MW01144776

THE LITTLE
DENTAL DRUG
BOOKLET

Handbook of Commonly Used
Dental Medications

2007-2008 Edition

Peter L. Jacobsen, PhD, DDS
Director

Oral Medicine Clinic
University of the Pacific
Arthur A. Dugoni School of Dentistry
2155 Webster St.
San Francisco, CA 94115
pgjacobs@pacbell.net
www.peterjacobsen.com

To place an order, call 1-866-397-3433
or visit www.lexi.com/lddb

NOTICE

This booklet is intended to serve the user as a handy reference and not as a complete drug information resource. Drug information is constantly evolving because of ongoing research and clinical experience and is often subject to interpretation. While great care has been taken to ensure the accuracy of the information presented, the reader is advised that the authors, editors, reviewers, and publishers cannot be responsible for the continued currency of the information or for any errors, omissions, or the application of this information, or for any consequences arising therefrom. Therefore, the author(s) and/or the publisher shall have no liability to any person or entity with regard to claims, loss, or damage caused, or alleged to be caused, directly or indirectly, by the use of information contained herein. Because of the dynamic nature of drug information, readers are advised that decisions regarding drug therapy must be based on the independent judgment of the clinician, changing information about a drug (eg, as reflected in the literature and manufacturer's most current product information), and changing medical practices.

The editors, authors, and contributors have written this book in their private capacities. No official support or endorsement by any federal or state agency, organization, or pharmaceutical company is intended or inferred.

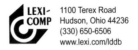

1100 Terex Road
Hudson, Ohio 44236
(330) 650-6506
www.lexi.com/lddb

ISBN: 978-1-59195-222-0

CONTENTS

SUBJECT INDEX

DRUG INDEX

DRUG INDEX

DRUG INDEX

SECTION I

PRESCRIPTION WRITING

Doctor's Name

Address

Phone Number

Patient's Name   Date

Patient's Address   Age

Rx   Drug Name   Dosage/Size

Disp   Number of tablets, capsules, ounces to be dispensed.
            (Roman numerals may be added as precaution for
            commonly abused drugs).

Sig   Direction on how drug is to be taken.

            Doctor's Signature
            State License Number
            DEA Number (if required)

Fill Generic: (This note, if appropriate, added to the prescription,
               allows the pharmacist to fill with the least expensive
               generic drug available.)

PRESCRIPTION REQUIREMENTS

1) Date

2) Full name and address of patient

3) Name and address of prescriber

4) Signature of prescriber

If Class II, III, IV drug, a Drug Enforcement Agency (DEA) number is necessary.

If a DEA Class II-V drug, in the state of California and several other states, a special tamper-proof prescription form printed only by state-approved printers is required. Check with your state dental society for details and contact information for authorized printers. Note, this form can be used for all prescriptions.

USEFUL INTERNET WEB SITES

www.ada.org
> the mothership of dentally-useful information

www.americanheart.org
> all guidelines are listed under "scientific statements"

www.dental.pacific.edu
> under "dental professional," guidelines for the dental management of medically-complex patients, and for HIV-infected patients, and health history translations

www.lexi.com/lddb
> website to order the current Little Dental Drug Booklet

COMMON ABBREVIATIONS

i, ii, iii	one, two, three
q	every (as in "every" 6 hours)
d	day
h	hours
prn	as needed
stat	right away, immediately
b	twice
t	three
q	four (same symbol denotes "every")

Example: t.i.d. = 3 times a day
q8h = every 8 hours

IF IN DOUBT, WRITE IT OUT!

SECTION II

Situations and the Appropriate Medications to Be Used

NOTES

1) ANXIETY CONTROL/ ANXIOLYSIS

Valium

Ativan

Halcion

Vistaril

Sonata

NOTE:

Anxiolysis, the decrease of anxiety in a fully alert and responsive patient, requires no permit.

Sedation, the mental and physiological slowing of the patient with medication may require a special permit in some states depending on the age of the patient and the level of sedation. If you intend to use medication to sedate a patient, you should acquire training and certification in such procedures.

In California, and possibly other states (check your state law), to give oral sedation to a child <13 years of age requires a special oral sedation permit from the State Board of Dental Examiners. Oral sedation means anything given by mouth that will sedate or relax the child. This would include sedative/ hypnotics (barbiturates, benzodiazepines), antihistamines, narcotics, and chloral hydrate.

MEDICATIONS: ANXIETY CONTROL/ANXIOLYSIS

Rx	**Valium 5 mg**
Disp	4 tablets
Sig	Take 1 tablet in evening before going to bed and 1 tablet 1 hour before your appointment

CAUTION:	Patient should not drive themselves to or from the appointment. Do not prescribe to pregnant women.
INGREDIENT:	Diazepam
NOTE:	Half-life: 20-100 hours

Rx	**Ativan 1 mg**
Disp	8 tablets
Sig	Take 2 tablets in evening before going to bed and 2 tablets 1 hour before your appointment

CAUTION:	(As for Valium)
INGREDIENT:	Lorazepam
NOTE:	Half-life: 12-14 hours

MEDICATIONS: ANXIETY CONTROL/ANXIOLYSIS

Rx   **Halcion 0.25 mg**

Disp   4 tablets

Sig   Take 1 tablet in evening before going to bed and 1 tablet 1 hour
before your appointment

CAUTION: (As for Valium)
INGREDIENT: Triazolam
NOTE: Half-life: 2-3 hours

Rx   **Vistaril 25 mg**

Disp   8 capsules

Sig   Take 2 capsules in evening before going to bed and 2 capsules
1 hour before your appointment

NOTE: Children's dosage is 1 tablet before bed and 1
tablet before appointment.
INGREDIENT: Hydroxyzine

Rx   **Sonata 5 mg**

Disp   8 tablets

Sig   Take 2 tablets at bedtime to assist in falling asleep and 2 tablets
1 hour before your appointment

INGREDIENT: Zaleplon
NOTE: Half-life: 1-2 hours

NOTES

2) PAIN

Mild Aspirin
Aleve
Celebrex
Ibuprofen
Dolobid
Acetaminophen

Moderate ASA Codeine
Synalgos DC
Ultracet
Lortab
Vicodin / Vicoprofen

Severe Percodan / Percocet
Combunox
Demerol
Dilaudid

All prescription narcotic pain medications can be filled generically, except Ultracet, Combunox, and Vicoprofen.

PAIN MANAGEMENT DECISION MAKING

Most pain in dentistry is in the "mild-to-moderate" range. The best pain control medication should be effective with a minimum risk for side effects or abuse.

ASPIRIN TOLERANT:

Ibuprofen
600 mg 4 times a day
(breakfast, lunch, dinner, and before bed)

(Start medication at time of the procedure and use for next several days to prevent pain from starting (preemptive analgesia). Ibuprofen is a very effective pain medicaiton, especially for inflammatory / dental pain.)

If pain is not controlled, switch to:

Vicodin or **Ultracet**

Even more effective, alternate whichever of these two drugs you choose with ibuprofen every 2 hours - for example, the patient is taking either:

Ibuprofen or **Vicodin / Ultracet** every 2 hours

If pain is very severe (ie, dry socket or equivalent), consider:

Percodan for several days, then back to the less powerful drugs.

ASPIRIN ALLERGIC:

Acetaminophen (OTC)
650-1000 mg 4 times a day

If pain is not controlled, stop Acetaminophen and switch to:

Tylenol #3, Vicodin, or **Ultracet**

If pain is very severe (ie, dry socket or equivalent), consider:

Percocet for several days, then back to the less powerful drugs.

MEDICATIONS: PAIN (MILD) OTC
Available over-the-counter (OTC)
Nonsteroidal and anti-inflammatory drugs (NSAIDs)

Rx   **Aspirin 325 mg (OTC)**

Disp

Sig   2-3 tablets every 4 hours

       NOTE: See Note 2 under Ibuprofen - it applies to all NSAIDs including aspirin.

Rx   **Ibuprofen 200 mg (OTC)**

Disp

Sig   2-3 tablets every 4 hours [maximum of 16 tablets (3200 mg) per day]

       NOTE 1:   Ibuprofen is available over-the-counter as Motrin, Advil, Nuprin, and many other brands in 200 mg tablets.

       NOTE 2:   a) NSAIDs should never be taken together, nor combined with aspirin. NSAIDs have antiinflammatory effects as well as producing analgesia.

                      b) An allergy to aspirin constitutes a contraindication to all NSAIDs.

                      c) Aspirin and the NSAIDs may increase post-treatment bleeding and GI bleeding.

MEDICATIONS: PAIN (MILD) OTC
Available over-the-counter (OTC)
Nonsteroidal and anti-inflammatory drugs (NSAIDs)

Rx   **Aleve (OTC)**

Disp

Sig   Take 2 tablets to start, then take 1 tablet every 6-12 hours up to 3 tablets (825 mg) per day

    INGREDIENT: Naproxen sodium 220 mg/tablet

    NOTE: 1) See Note 2 under Ibuprofen (previous page). It applies to all NSAIDs.

                 2) Aleve and Anaprox are the same drug. OTC dosage is lower, duration is longer, interval between dose longer per FDA rule.

MEDICATIONS: PAIN (MILD) OTC
Available over-the-counter (OTC)
(For patients allergic to aspirin and other NSAIDs)

Rx   **Acetaminophen 325 mg (OTC)**

Disp

Sig   Take 2-3 tablets every 4 hours

    PRODUCTS
    INCLUDE: Tylenol, Datril, Anacin 3, and many others

    NOTE: Acetaminophen can be given if patient has allergy, bleeding problems, or stomach upset secondary to aspirin or NSAIDs.

MEDICATIONS: PAIN (MILD) Rx
Require Prescription (Rx)
Nonsteroidal anti-inflammatory drugs (NSAIDs)

Rx*	**Motrin 600 mg**

Disp   28 tablets

Sig   Take 1 tablet 3 times per day

INGREDIENT: Ibuprofen

NOTE: For severe pain, Motrin (600 mg) can be given up to 4 times per day.

Rx*	**Dolobid 500 mg**

Disp   16 tablets

Sig   Take 2 tablets initially then 1 tablet every 8-12 hours for pain

INGREDIENT: Diflunisal

MEDICATIONS: PAIN (MILD) Rx
Require Prescription (Rx)

Rx*	**Anaprox**

Disp | 16 tablets

Sig | Take 2 tablets to start, then take 1 tablet every 6-8 hours, not to exceed 5 tablets (1375 mg) in 24 hours

INGREDIENT: Naproxen sodium 275 mg/tablet

NOTE: This is the prescription form of Aleve

---

*NOTE: All of the above drugs are NSAIDs. See Note 2 under Ibuprofen (pg 21) - it applies to all NSAIDs.

*NOTE: All Rx NSAIDs can be taken with food to minimize risk of stomach upset.

Rx	**Celebrex 200 mg**

Disp | 15 capsules

Sig | Take 2 capsules stat, then 1 capsule every 12 hours

INGREDIENT: Celecoxib

NOTE: Celebrex is a sulfa drug and should not be given to patients allergic to sulfa drugs.

NOTE: Prolonged use (which seldom, if ever, occurs in dental settings), may increase the risk of cardiovascular events.

MEDICATIONS: PAIN (MODERATE)
All narcotics are "scheduled" and require DEA license to prescribe, except Ultracet.

The following is a guideline to use when prescribing codeine with either aspirin or acetaminophen (Tylenol):

Codeine No. 2 = Codeine 15 mg
Codeine No. 3 = Codeine 30 mg
Codeine No. 4 = Codeine 60 mg

EXAMPLE: ASA No. 3 = aspirin 325 mg + codeine 30 mg

Rx	**Tylenol #3**
Disp	28 tablets
Sig	Take 1-2 tablets every 4 hours as needed for pain

	INGREDIENTS:	Acetaminophen 300 mg; Codeine 30 mg
	NOTE:	For pediatric liquid preparation, see pages 65-67 under Pediatric Dosages.
	SCHEDULE	III

NOTE: All of the above can be filled generically.

MEDICATIONS: PAIN (MODERATE)

Rx	**Synalgos DC**

Disp   28 capsules

Sig   Take 1-2 capsules every 4 hours as needed for pain

INGREDIENTS:	Dihydrocodeine 16 mg; Aspirin 356.4 mg; Caffeine 30 mg
SCHEDULE:	III

Rx	**Vicoprofen**

Disp   16 tablets

Sig   Take 1-2 tablets every 4-6 hours as needed for pain

INGREDIENTS:	Hydrocodone 7.5 mg; Ibuprofen 200 mg
SCHEDULE:	III

Rx	**Vicodin (or select brand below)**

Disp   16 tablets

Sig   Take 1-2 tablets every 4-6 hours as needed for pain

INGREDIENTS:	Hydrocodone 5 mg; Acetaminophen 500 mg
OTHER BRAND NAMES:	Lortab, Stagesic, Anexsia, Co-Gesic
SCHEDULE:	III

NOTE: All of the above can be filled generically, except Vicoprofen.

MEDICATIONS: PAIN (MODERATE)
(For patients allergic to aspirin and opioids)

Rx	**Ultracet**
Disp	36 tablets
Sig	Take 2 tablets every 4-6 hours (do not exceed 8 tablets in 24 hours)

INGREDIENTS: Acetaminophen 325 mg; Tramadol 37.5 mg
SCHEDULE: None

MEDICATIONS: PAIN (SEVERE)
All narcotics are "scheduled" and require DEA license to prescribe, except Ultracet

Rx	**Demerol 50 mg**
Disp	16 tablets
Sig	Take 1 tablet every 4 hours for pain

INGREDIENTS: Meperidine
SCHEDULE: II

Rx*	**Dilaudid 2 mg**
Disp	16 tablets
Sig	Take 1 tablet every 4 hours for pain

INGREDIENTS: Hydromorphone
SCHEDULE: II

NOTE: All of the above can be filled generically, except Ultracet

MEDICATIONS: PAIN (SEVERE)

Rx   **Percodan**

Disp   20 tablets

Sig   Take 1-2 tablets every 4 hours for pain

INGREDIENTS: Oxycodone 4.88 mg; Aspirin 325 mg
SCHEDULE: II

Rx   **Percocet 5 mg** (or select brand below)

Disp   20 tablets

Sig   Take 1-2 tablets every 4-6 hours for pain

INGREDIENTS: Oxycodone 5 mg; Acetaminophen 325 mg
SCHEDULE: II
OTHER BRAND
NAMES: Roxicet, Tylox

Rx   **Combunox**

Disp   16 tablets

Sig   Take 1 tablet every 6 hours for pain

INGREDIENTS: Oxycodone 5 mg; Ibuprofen 400 mg
SCHEDULE: II

NOTE: All of the above can be filled generically, except Combunox

3) INFECTION (Bacterial)

Amoxicillin
Augmentin
Azithromycin (Zithromax)
Cephalexin
Clindamycin (Cleocin)
Dicloxacillin
Erythromycin
Metronidazole (Flagyl)
Penicillin VK

ANTIBIOTIC DECISION MAKING

1. Drugs of choice for dental infections:

   Penicillin or **Amoxicillin**

2. If no response in 48-72 hours then use:

   A. Clindamycin (best choice)

   or   **B. Cephalexin** or **Dicloxacillin**

   or   **C.** Some dentists elect to add **Metronidazole** to the **Amoxicillin**

3. If no response to choice **B** or **C** in 24-48 hours, then use:

   Clindamycin

   (Be sure to incise and drain, if appropriate)

IF PATIENT IS ALLERGIC TO PENICILLIN

1. First drug of choice is:

   Clindamycin

2. If no response in 48-72 hours, then use:

   Azithromycin (Zithromax)

(If no response to above protocol, refer to or consult with an oral surgeon, endodontist, or infectious disease physician)

(See page 63 for sinus infections)

MEDICATIONS: INFECTION (BACTERIAL)*

Rx	**Amoxicillin 500 mg**
Disp	30 tablets
Sig	Take 1 tablet 3 times per day

Rx	**Augmentin 500 mg**
Disp	30 tablets
Sig	Take 1 tablet 3 times per day

INGREDIENTS: Amoxicillin 500 mg; Clavulanate Potassium
NOTE: Augmentin is amoxicillin protected from penicillinase by clavulanate.

Rx	**Cephalexin 500 mg**
Disp	40 capsules
Sig	Take 1 capsule 4 times per day

Rx	**Clindamycin 150 mg**
Disp	40 capsules
Sig	Take 2 capsules every 6 hours

NOTE: All antibiotics have risk of pseudomembranous colitis, especially clindamycin.

*For pediatric dosage, see pages 65-67.

MEDICATIONS: INFECTION (BACTERIAL)*

Rx	**Dicloxacillin 500 mg**
Disp	40 capsules
Sig	Take 1 capsule every 6 hours

Rx	**Erythromycin Base 250 mg**
Disp	40 tablets (enteric coated)
Sig	Take 1 tablet 4 times per day
	NOTE: Erythromycin has a high risk for drug-drug interactions and stomach upset. Also risk of cardiac problems.

Rx	**Metronidazole 500 mg**
Disp	40 tablets
Sig	Take 1 tablet 4 times per day

Rx	**Penicillin VK 500 mg**
Disp	40 tablets
Sig	Take 1 tablet 4 times per day

Rx	**Zithromax (Z-pak)**
Disp	1 pack (6 x 250 mg tablets)
Sig	Take 2 tablets on day 1 and 1 tablet on days 2-5
	INGREDIENT: Azithromycin

*For pediatric dosage see pages 65-67.

4) INFECTION (Fungal)

Nystatin Oral Suspension
Nystatin Tablets
Nystatin Ointment or Cream
Nystatin Powder
Mycelex
Nizoral
Diflucan

ANTIFUNGAL DECISION MAKING

DRUGS OF CHOICE FOR ORAL FUNGAL INFECTIONS*

The first drugs of choice for local treatment of oral fungal infections are:

Mycelex Troche or **Nystatin Tablets**

The drug of choice for systematic treatment of oral fungal infections is:

Diflucan

The drug of choice for angular cheilitis is:

Mycolog II Cream (Rx on page 50)

NOTE: Chlorhexidine (Rx on page 58) has been shown to be of value to
control oral fungal infections, especially in HIV-infected patients.
(Symptomatic patients rinse 2 times per day; asymptomatic
patients rinse 1 time per day at night.)

* Pediatric dosages are on pages 65-67.

MEDICATIONS: INFECTION (FUNGAL)

Rx   **Mycelex Troche 10 mg**

Disp   70 troches

Sig   Dissolve 1 troche in mouth 5 times per day

     INGREDIENTS: Clotrimazole

     NOTE: The troche contains sucrose, risk of caries with prolonged use (>3 months).

Rx   **Nystatin Tablets**

Disp   30 tablets

Sig   Dissolve 1 tablet in mouth until gone, 3 times per day

     INGREDIENTS: 100,000 units of nystatin per tablet

     SPECIAL INDICATIONS: The soluble tablet is more effective than an oral suspension, but is sometimes hard to find.

MEDICATIONS: INFECTION (FUNGAL)

Rx	**Nystatin Oral Suspension**

Disp   300 mL

Sig   Use 1 teaspoonful for 2 minutes 4-5 times per day then spit out

INGREDIENTS: Nystatin 100,000 units/mL. Vehicle contains 50% sucrose and not more than 1% alcohol. High risk of dental decay with prolonged use (>3 months).

Rx	**Nystatin** (Ointment, Cream, or Powder - select one)

Disp   15 g or 30 g tube

Sig   Apply liberally to affected areas 3 times per day

INGREDIENTS:

Cream:	100,000 units nystatin per gram, aqueous vanishing cream base.
Ointment:	100,000 units nystatin per gram, polyethylene and mineral oil gel base.
Powder:	5,000 units nystatin per mg. May be sprinkled into dentures.

Rx   **Diflucan 100 mg**

Disp   16 tablets

Sig   Take 2 tablets the first day and 1 tablet each day thereafter until resolved

INGREDIENT: Fluconazole

NOTE: To be used if *Candida* infection does not respond to local oral drug.

Rx   **Nizoral 200 mg**

Disp   10 tablets

Sig   Take 1 tablet per day

INGREDIENT: Ketoconazole

NOTE: High risk of multiple severe drug interactions. Check with pharmacist about interactions if patient is taking other medications.

NOTE: To be used if *Candida* infection does not respond to local oral drugs.

NOTE: Potential for liver toxicity. Liver function should be monitored with long-term use (>3 weeks).

NOTES

5) INFECTION (Viral)

Abreva
Denavir
Valtrex
Xylocaine 2% Viscous
Zovirax
Zovirax Ointment 5%

HERPES SIMPLEX MANAGEMENT

Oral herpes simplex is a viral disease. Secondary attacks occur primarily on lips, but when they occur inside the mouth, they occur as clusters of pinpoint ulcers only on attached (overlying bone) mucosa.

PRIMARY ATTACK

- **Xylocaine 2% Viscous** (palliative)
- **Valacyclovir** (Valtrex®)
- Fluids and liquid food supplements

SECONDARY ATTACK

- **Valacyclovir** at first indication of attack
- May supplement with **Acyclovir** (Zovirax®) ointment or **Penciclovir** (Denavir®) or **Docosanol** (Abreva®) as needed.

PROPHYLAXIS: ACUTE

- **Valacyclovir**, 1 day prior, day of, and 2 days after precipitating event (eg, sun exposure, dental visit)

PROPHYLAXIS: CHRONIC (for severe cases)

- **Famciclovir**, 250 mg, 2 times per day for a year
  or
- **Valacyclovir**, 1 tablet 2 times per day for a year

  Re-evaluate need for prophylaxis yearly by discontinuing drug and observing the patient for recurrence.

MEDICATIONS: INFECTION (VIRAL)

Rx	**Xylocaine 2% Viscous**

Disp   100 mL or 450 mL

Sig   Use 2 teaspoonsful to rinse around oral cavity as needed to relieve pain - spit out

INGREDIENT: Lidocaine HCl

Rx	**Zovirax 200 mg**

Disp   50-60 capsules

Sig   Take 1 capsule 5 times per day for 10 days or 2 capsules 3 times per day for 10 days

INGREDIENT: Acyclovir

Rx	**Zovirax Ointment 5%**

Disp   15 g

Sig   Apply thin layer to lesion 6 times per day for 7 days

INGREDIENT: Acyclovir

Rx	**Denavir**

Disp   1.5 g

Sig   Apply every 2 hours during waking hours for a period of 4 days

INGREDIENT: Penciclovir 1%

MEDICATIONS: INFECTION (VIRAL)

Rx   **Valtrex 500 mg**

Disp   8 tablets

Sig   Take 4 tablets at first sign of attack and then take 4 tablets 12 hours later

        INGREDIENT: Valacyclovir

        NOTE: Not for HIV patients; may cause thrombocytopenia.

Rx   **Abreva (OTC)**

Disp   2 g

Sig   Apply to lesion 5 times per day until lesion is gone

        INGREDIENT: Docosanol 10%

Rx   **Viroxyn** (Available through DDS office or online)

Disp   1 tube

Sig   Break the tube, rub ulcer/starting herpes lesion with fluid until it stings. Discard tube. Repeat once 12 hours later, if needed.

        NOTE: Viroxyn can be obtained at www.viroxyn.com.

6) ORAL SOFT TISSUE PROBLEMS

Aphthous	Benadryl/Kaopectate
	Lidex Ointment
	Kenalog in Orabase
	Dexamethasone Elixir
Necrotizing Ulcerative Gingivitis	Betadine
Allergy	Benadryl
Oral Inflammatory Disease	Lidex Ointment
	Kenalog in Orabase
	Prednisone
	Temovate Ointment
	Dexamethasone Elixir
Angular Cheilitis	Mycolog II Cream

APHTHOUS ULCERS (CANKER SORES) MANAGEMENT

Aphthous is an autoimmune disease with poorly understood triggering causes. The lesions occur exclusively on <u>unattached</u> (cheek, floor of mouth, etc) mucosa. (As opposed to secondary herpes simplex, which, intraorally, occurs only on <u>attached</u> mucosa.)

Treatment for canker sores is divided into 3 sections:

1. Prevention
2. Pain relief
3. Pharmacological treatment

PREVENTION

Avoid triggering foods:
Nuts, chocolate, acidic fruits

Avoid trauma:
Toothbrush trauma, cheek bite, etc

Avoid stress:
Now that is useless advice... who has the time to avoid stress?

Avoid sodium and lauryl sulfate:
A soap found in most toothpaste and mouthwashes. Consider Biotene toothpaste or Rembrandt for canker sore sufferers.

Consider an antimicrobial mouthrinse:
Chlorhexidine (Rx on page 58) or **Listerine.** For prevention only. Do not prescribe for treatment - it does not work and the alcohol stings.

APHTHOUS ULCERS (CANKER SORES) MANAGEMENT

PAIN RELIEF

Products which coat the lesion or numb the ulcers or both:

Coat and numb lesion:
> **Orabase B**
> **Zilactin B**
> **Kanka**

Coat lesion only:
> **Orabase Soothe-n-Seal**
> **Liquid Carafate**
> **Benadryl / Kaopectate** (Rx on page 47)

PHARMACOLOGICAL TREATMENT

Corticosteroids to reverse the autoimmune process (all are by prescription):

> **Kenalog in Orabase** (often not potent enough) (Rx page 48)

> **Lidex ointment** (Rx page 48)

> **Temovate ointment** (Rx page 48)

> **Dexamethasone elixir** (Rx page 48)

On rare occasions:
> **Prednisone**, 40 mg/day for 7 days (Rx page 49)

CAUTERIZING TREATMENT:

> **Debacterol** (Rx page 49)
> **Ora 5** (www.ora5.com, 1-800-746-5486)

(ACUTE) NECROTIZING ULCERATING GINGIVITIS (ANUG OR NUG)

NUG is a specific bacterial (spirochetal) infection.

TREATMENT STEPS:

1. **Amoxicillin** to treat infection (Rx page 31)

2. **Chlorhexidine** (Rx page 58) or **Betadine** to aid in treating infection

3. **Hydrogen peroxide** rinse and/or warm saline rinse

4. Short term pain medication as needed (Rx page 21)

5. Dental cleaning when patient is comfortable.

Rx	**Betadine Solution**
Disp	8 oz
Sig	Rinse 1 teaspoonful in mouth for 1 minute and spit out, 2 times per day

INGREDIENT:	Povidone-iodine 10%
NOTE:	Not to be used in patients allergic to iodine. Solution should be completely spit out.
NOTE:	For short-term use only, maximum 2 days.
NOTE:	For anticaries use see page 54.

MEDICATIONS: ORAL ALLERGY

Rx	**Benadryl 50 mg**
Disp	16 capsules
Sig	3-4 times per day

INGREDIENTS:	Diphenhydramine hydrochloride
SPECIAL INDICATIONS:	Use 3-4 times per day for 4 days depending on duration of allergic reaction.

Rx	**Benadryl Syrup (Mix 50/50) with Kaopectate**
Disp	8 oz total
Sig	Rinse 1 tablespoonful in mouth for 1 minute as needed to relieve pain or burning, then spit out

MEDICATIONS: ORAL INFLAMMATORY DISEASE

Rx	**Lidex Ointment**
Disp	15 g
Sig	Apply thin layer to oral lesions 4-6 times per day
	INGREDIENT: Fluocinonide 0.05%

Rx	**Temovate Ointment**
Disp	15 g
Sig	Apply thin layer to oral lesions 4-6 times per day
	INGREDIENT: Clobetasol 0.05%

Rx	**Kenalog in Orabase**
Disp	5 g
Sig	Apply thin layer to affected area 3 times per day
	NOTE: If stronger corticosteroid is needed, use Lidex

Rx	**Dexamethasone Elixir**
Disp	500 mL
Sig	Rinse 1 teaspoonful in mouth for 1 minute, 4-5 times per day, then spit out
	INGREDIENT: Dexamethasone 0.5 mg/5 mL

MEDICATIONS: ORAL INFLAMMATORY DISEASE

Rx   **Prednisone 5 mg**

Disp   40 tablets

Sig   Take 4 tablets in AM and 4 tablets at noon for 5 days

        CAUTION: 1. Take medication with food

                       2. Use with extreme caution. This is a potent systemic dosage. Consult with patient's physician, an oral medicine DDS (at dental schools), or medical textbook if questions on dosage, indications, or contraindications arise.

MEDICATIONS: APHTHOUS (CAUTERIZER)

Rx   **Debacterol** (Available through DDS office)

Disp   1 tube

Sig   Break internal glass tube, touch saturated cotton tip to ulcer (warn patient, it will hurt). Hold in place for 20-30 seconds.

        NOTE: Debacterol can be obtained at www.epien.com under "products", 1-888-884-4675, or from most dental supply companies.

ANGULAR CHEILITIS
(CRACKING IN THE CORNER OF THE MOUTH)

Rx	**Mycolog II Cream**
Disp	15 g
Sig	Apply to corners of mouth 4 times per day

INGREDIENTS: 100,000 units nystatin per gram
1 mg triamcinolone acetonide

7) MISCELLANEOUS

Dentin Hypersensitivity Treatment*

Tooth Whitening Products*

Anticaries Agents*

Antigingivitis / Antiplaque Agents*

**Necrotizing Ulcerating Periodontitis
(HIV Periodontal Disease)**

Saliva Problems

Sinus Infection Treatment

Pediatric Dosages

*NOTE: Check www.ada.org/public for most
current list of over-the-counter products
that have the ADA Seal of Acceptance.

DENTIN HYPERSENSITIVITY

SUGGESTED STEPS IN RESOLVING DENTIN HYPERSENSITIVITY:

A thorough exam to rule out any other source for the problem such as tooth fracture, occlusal trauma, or irreversible pulpitis, must be done first. The most common reason for persistent hypersensitivity is bruxing.

TREATMENT STEPS:

Step 1. Home treatment with a desensitizing toothpaste containing potassium nitrate (used to brush teeth at least 2 times per day, as well as a thin layer applied to affected teeth and left overnight, each night for 3-4 weeks). Tell patient not to use tartar control toothpaste. It may slow natural occlusion of dentinal tubules by preventing calcium precipitation.

Step 2. In office, **SootheRx** by Omnii or potassium oxalate application (**ThermaTrol** by Premier) or a fluoride varnish such as **CavityShield**, **Duraphat**, or **VarnishAmerica**.

Step 3. If sensitivity still not tolerable to patient, consider pumice then seal teeth with dentin adhesive (ie, **Amalgabond** or **All-bond**). If still sensitive, consider composite or composite/glass ionomer restoration.

DENTIN HYPERSENSITIVITY

HOME USE PRODUCTS (OTC)

Potassium nitrate is the active ingredient in almost all ADA-accepted desensitizing toothpastes. (**Crest Sensitivity Protection**, **Sensodyne**, **Colgate Sensitive**, **Oragel Sensitive**, etc). **Crest ProHealth** contains stannous fluoride.

OTHER HOME USE PRODUCTS

Stannous fluoride formulations (usually less effective than potassium nitrate for dentin hypersensitivity) (**Gel-Kam Gel**, **Stop Gel**, or any stannous fluoride gel. Some practitioners have gotten good results with Rx sodium fluoride (5000 ppm) (Rx pages 56-57).

TOOTH WHITENING PRODUCTS

Most dental whitening products accepted by the ADA contain some type of peroxide, which oxidizes the stains. These accepted products must be prescribed/dispensed by a dentist. Crest White Strips are an effective OTC, peroxide-containing whitening product.

To date, several OTC toothpastes, **Crest ProHealth**, **Crest Extra Whitening**, **Crest Multicare Whitening Toothpaste**, **Colgate Total Plus**, etc, have the ADA seal for whitening. The main mechanism is abrasive removal of stains.

ANTICARIES AGENTS

MANAGING DENTAL DECAY AS AN INFECTIOUS DISEASE

Compounds used to kill cariogenic bacteria *(for optimal control of patients with high decay rate):*

- CHLORHEXIDINE: Chlorhexidine (0.12%) Oral Rinse (page 58), 2 times per day for 2 weeks, every 3 months

or

- IODINE: (Be sure patient does not have iodine allergy). Rinse 1 teaspoon of **Betadine®** (povidone-iodine 10%) in mouth for 1 minute every 2 months. (I know it tastes awful, get over it!)

plus

- XYLITOL: Xylitol is a natural sugar that cariogenic bacteria cannot metabolize into tooth dissolving acidic by-products. It's presence alters the oral bacterial environment and decreases the risk of decay.

  DOSAGE: Chew 2 sticks of gum for 5 minutes, 4-5 times/day (discontinue use if TMJ symptoms occur) or suck on xylitol candy 4-5 times/day.

  NOTE: Xylitol should be used after the chlorhexidine or iodine rinses over the next 3 months. The rinses kill the cariogenic organisms and the xylitol creates the optimal environment for oral repopulation with noncariogenic organisms.

  SOURCES: www.xylitolstore.com 1-877-239-8910
  www.omnipharma.com 1-800-445-3386
  www.xlear.com 1-877-332-1001

ANTICARIES AGENTS

Fluorides to "harden" tooth structure:

> Of course, OTC toothpaste (1000-1500 ppm)
> and, consider OTC fluoride rinses (230 ppm)

High Caries Rate:

> Rx: Sodium fluoride (5000 ppm) gel or toothpaste
> and
> Fluoride varnish (22,600 ppm) applied every 6 months

FLUORIDE: PRESCRIPTION SYSTEMIC

Rx	**Sodium Fluoride Tablets** (size based on table below)

Disp   120

Sig   Chew and dissolve 1 tablet in mouth, then swallow, once per day, preferably before bedtime after brushing

> NOTE: Chewing and dissolving fluoride in mouth is
> very important. Much, if not all, of the systemic
> fluoride tablet benefit is topical.

ADA Recommended Supplemental Fluoride Dosage Schedule

Age (years)	Concentration of fluoride ion in drinking water (PPM)		
	<0.3	**0.3-0.6**	**>0.6**
6 mo to 3 y	0.25 mg	0	0
3 to 6 y	0.50 mg	0.25 mg	0
6 to 16 y	1 mg	0.50 mg	0

ANTICARIES AGENTS

FLUORIDE: PRESCRIPTION TOPICAL

Rx	**Neutral Sodium Fluoride Gel / Toothpaste 1.1 (5000 ppm)**

Disp	2 oz

Sig	Brush on teeth if paste or place 1 teaspoonful of gel in fluoride tray and apply to teeth 3-5 minutes, or while you are in the shower, once per day

COMMERCIAL PRODUCTS:

ControlRx (Omnii Products)

Neutracare Home Topical (Oral-B)

Prevident Gel or toothpaste (Colgate)

NOTE: If caries severe, after brushing teeth, use neutral fluoride gel (5000 ppm) in custom tray for 3-5 minutes, once per day, for as long as needed (years).

Rx	**Fluoride Varnish** (22,600 ppm F)

COMMERCIAL PRODUCTS FOR DENTAL OFFICE:

CavityShield (www.omniipharma.com)

Duraphat (Colgate)

VarnishAmerica (1-800-523-0191)

(www.medicalproductslaboratories.com)

ANTICARIES AGENTS

FLUORIDE: NONPRESCRIPTION TOPICAL

Rx   Any **ADA-Approved Toothpaste** (1000-1500 ppm)

Rx   **OTC Fluoride Rinses** (230 ppm F)

      COMMERCIAL PRODUCTS:
          ACT Fluoride Rinse (Johnson & Johnson)
          Fluorigard (Colgate)

Rx   **Stannous Fluoride 0.4%** (Brush on Gel) (1500 ppm)

Disp   4 oz

Sig   Brush on teeth or place 1 teaspoon in fluoride tray and apply to teeth for 3-5 minutes once per day.

      COMMERCIAL PRODUCTS:
          Gel-Kam Gel (Colgate)
          PerioMed (Omnii Products)
          Stop Gel (Oral-B)

      NOTE: For rampant decay in children, <u>very small amounts</u> of stannous fluoride (1500 ppm) may be <u>dabbed on lesion</u> daily by parent to arrest decay until definitive treatment can be rendered. Prolonged use would increase risk of fluorosis.

ADA ACCEPTED ANTIPLAQUE AND ANTIGINGIVITIS AGENTS

Rx	**Chlorhexidine Oral Rinse 0.12%**
Disp	3 x 16 oz
Sig	1/2 oz swish for 30 seconds 2 times per day

CAUTION: Chlorhexidine may:
- stain teeth yellow to brown
- alter taste (temporary)
- increase the deposition of calculus
- and requires a prescription
  (other than that, it is excellent)

NOTE: Peridex, PerioGard, and other brands

NOTE: Also, consider for patients with high decay rate (see page 48).

Rx	**Listerine (OTC)**
Disp	
Sig	Rinse 1 tablespoon in mouth for 30 seconds, 2 times per day

Rx	**Crest ProHealth Toothpaste or Colgate Total Toothpaste (OTC)**
Disp	
Sig	Brush teeth with toothpaste 2-3 times per day

MANAGEMENT OF NECROTIZING ULCERATING PERIODONTITIS
(HIV-Associated Periodontal Disease)

INITIAL TREATMENT (IN-OFFICE)

- Betadine Rinse (page 46)

  NOTE: Ensure patient has no iodine allergies

- Gentle debridement / dental cleaning

AT-HOME

- Chlorhexidine rinse (page 58)

- Metronidazole (Flagyl) 7-10 days (page 32)

FOLLOW-UP THERAPY

- Proper dental cleaning including scaling and root planing (repeat as needed)

- Continue Chlorhexidine rinse as needed

  NOTE: Most patients respond well to therapy and only normal oral hygiene and cleaning are needed.

SALIVARY HYPOSECRETION / XEROSTOMIA

Dry mouth is most commonly a side effect of medications, but can be caused by radiation (cancer treatment) or immunologic (Sjögren's Syndrome) destruction of the salivary glands. Advanced age can also lead to decreased resting levels of saliva production, though stimulated flows are usually normal.

TREATMENT: If salivary glands are still functional, they can be stimulated with pilocarpine or cevimeline.

Rx	**Salagen 5 mg**
Disp	90 tablets
Sig	Take 1 tablet 3-4 times per day (maximum dose: 10 mg 3 times per day)

	INGREDIENT:	Pilocarpine hydrochloride
	NOTE:	Pilocarpine is available as a generic
	CAUTION:	Read prescribing information. Many contra-indications (ie, glaucoma) and precautions (eye, heart, lung, etc, diseases)

Rx	**Evoxac 30 mg**
Disp	90 tablets
Sig	Take 1 tablet 3 times per day

	INGREDIENT:	Cevimeline
	CAUTION:	Read prescribing information. Many contra-indications (ie, glaucoma) and precautions (eye, heart, lung, etc, diseases)

SALIVARY HYPOSECRETION / XEROSTOMIA

PALLIATIVE TREATMENT OF DRY MOUTH:

Artificial Lubricant:

Biotene Oral Balance Gel (Laclede)

Oralbalance Dry Mouth liquid moisturizer

(www.laclede.com, 1-800-922-5856)

Artificial Salivas:

Saliva substitute (Roxane)

MouthKote (Pasnell)

Moi-Stir (Kingswood)

Most people just use plain water in a small squirt bottle

Nonirritating Toothpaste

Biotene Toothpaste (Laclede)

Mouth Spray

Breathtech Plaque Fighter Mouth Spray

(www.omniipharma.com, 1-800-445-3386)

Salivart

Note: See "Managing Dental Decay" for those patients with severe xerostomia (pages 54-57)

SALIVARY HYPOSECRETION (SIALOSCHESIS)

The following two drugs are used to block excessive salivary flow during restorative procedures.

Rx	**Propantheline 15 mg**

Disp   # (1-2 tablets per appointment)

Sig   Take 1 tablet 30 minutes before dental appointment

     INGREDIENT: Propantheline

     NOTE: In some patients, 2 tablets may be needed.

     CAUTION: Contraindicated in glaucoma. Can dry eyes, so remove contact lenses.

Rx	**Atropine 0.4 mg**

Disp   # (1 tablet per appointment)

Sig   Take 1 tablet 1 hour before dental appointment on an empty stomach

     INGREDIENT: Atropine

     CAUTION: Contraindicated in glaucoma. Can dry eyes, so remove contact lenses.

SINUS INFECTION TREATMENT

DDS must elect to treat sinuses, but only to rule out dental problems, otherwise, refer to physician.

Rx	**Amoxicillin 500 mg**
Disp	21 tablets
Sig	Take 1 tablet 3 times per day

OR

Rx	**Augmentin 500 mg**
Disp	30
Sig	Take 1 tablet 3 times per day
	INGREDIENTS: Amoxicillin and Clavulanate Potassium

TREATMENT: The selected antibiotic (above) should be used with the compounds below to block the histamine effect (Claritin) and to shrink the sinuses (Neo-Synephrine).

Rx	**Claritin 10 mg (OTC)***
Disp	14 tablets
Sig	Take 1 tablet per day

Rx	**Neo-Synephrine 12 Hour (OTC)***
Disp	15 mL
Sig	2 sprays in each nostril, not more often than every 4 hours
	INGREDIENTS: Oxymetazoline
	OTHER BRANDS: Afrin, Vicks, Sinex

*OTC = over-the-counter

DRY SOCKET (ACUTE / ALVEOLAR OSTEITIS)

This is a necrosis of bone following a dental extraction. It is not an infection and usually not associated with an infection. Treatment is designed to soothe the pain while the area heals.

TREATMENT:

1. Gently irrigate socket with saline.

2. Gently fill socket site with **Alvogyl** (Septodont: 800-872-8305, www.septodontusa.com).

3. **Alvogyl** dissolves on its own, and does not need to be removed.

4. Repeat appplication if product is gone and pain persists.

NOTE: Prescribe pain medication as needed (pages 20-28).

NOTE: If obvious pus/infection, then it is not a dry socket, it is an infection and you must manage as an infection and prescribe antibiotics (pages 30-32).

PEDIATRIC DOSAGES

Pediatric dosages are given as mg of drug per kg (1 kg = 2.2 lbs) of child per 24 hours. The average child is considered an adult by age 12-14 depending on weight. **The child dose should never exceed the adult dose**, even if the calculation suggests it does.

The table on the following pages lists the <u>maximum dose in mg/kg (1 kg = 2.2 lbs) for a child in a 24-hour period</u>. It also indicates the frequency of dosing. Please note the maximum 24-hour dose must be divided by the suggested number of doses per 24 hours, to get the amount for each dose.

If there are any concerns or questions as to appropriateness of dosage, drug interactions, or indications for the drug, consult the child's physician, a pharmacist, or the drug's package insert information.

NOTE: In California, and possibly other states (check your state law), to
          give oral sedation to a child <13 years of age requires a special
          oral sedation permit from the State Board of Dental Examiners.
          Oral sedation means anything given by mouth that will sedate or
          relax the child. This would include sedative/hypnotics
          (barbiturates, benzodiazepines), antihistamines, narcotics, and
          chloral hydrate.

PEDIATRIC DOSAGES

Acetaminophen	12-16 mg/kg, 4x day max dose: 50-65 mg/kg/24 hr
Acetaminophen 125 mg + Codeine 12 mg/5 mL	3-7 y/o 1 teaspoon (5 mL) every 6 hr
Acetaminophen 125 mg + Codeine 12 mg/5 mL	8-12 y/o 2 teaspoons (10 mL) every 6 hr
Acyclovir	>2 y/o - same as adult
Amoxicillin	8-33 mg/kg, 3x day max dose: 25-100 mg/kg/24 hr
Cephalexin	20-25 mg/kg, 4x day max dose: 75-100 mg/kg/24 hr
Clindamycin	3-8 mg/kg, 3x day max dose: 10-25 mg/kg/24 hr
Clotrimazole	>2 y/o, same as adult Spit out saliva if stomach upset
Dicloxacillin	6-25 mg/kg, 4x day max dose: 25-100 mg/kg/24 hr
Diflucan	>3 y/o, 3-6 mg/kg/24 hr
Erythromycin	5-12 mg/kg, 4x day max dose: 20-50 mg/kg/24 hr

Ibuprofen	10 mg/kg, 4x day max dose: 40 mg/kg/24 hr
Ketoconazole	>2 y/o, same as adult
Metronidazole	12-18 mg/kg, 3x day max dose: 35-50 mg/kg/24 hr
Mycelex	>2 y/o, same as adult Spit out saliva if stomach upset
Naproxen sodium	5 mg/kg, 2x day max dose: 10 mg/kg/24 hr
Valium*	0.04-0.25 mg/kg, 3x day max dose: 0.12-0.8 mg/kg/24 hr *See Note, bottom page 65

NOTE: For pediatric doses for the prophylaxis of infectious (bacterial) endocarditis, see page 72.

NOTES

8) PROPHYLACTIC ANTIBIOTIC COVERAGE

Amoxicillin

Ampicillin

Azithromycin

Cefazolin

Ceftriaxone

Cephalexin

Clarithromycin

Clindamycin

PROPHYLACTIC ANTIBIOTIC COVERAGE FOR THE PREVENTION OF BACTERIAL ENDOCARDITIS

Current American Heart Association Guidelines
Published May 8, 2007, *Circulation*, Vol 115.

Cardiac Conditions for Which Prophylaxis for Dental Procedures is Recommended*

Prosthetic Cardiac Valve

Previous Infective Endocarditis

Congenital Heart Disease (CHD)

> Unrepaired cyanotic CHD, including palliative shunts and conduits

> Completely repaired congenital heart defect with prosthetic material or device, whether placed by surgery or by catheter intervention, during the first 6 months after the procedure (endothelialization occurs within 6 months of procedure)

> Repaired CHD with residual defects at the site or adjacent to the site of a prosthetic patch or prosthetic device (which inhibits endothelialization)

Cardiac transplant recipients who develop cardiac valvulopathy

---

If patient's physician requests prophylaxis for dental procedure, but patient does not meet ADA/AHA criteria for needing it, then physician should prescribe prophylaxis, patient takes it under their direction, and they come to you safe for dental procedures.

*Except for the cardiac conditions listed above, antibiotic prophylaxis is no longer recommended for any cardiac condition or problem.

PROPHYLACTIC ANTIBIOTIC COVERAGE FOR THE PREVENTION OF BACTERIAL ENDOCARDITIS

STANDARD REGIMEN

Rx	**Amoxicillin 500 mg**

Disp   4 tablets

Sig   Take 4 tablets (2 g) 30-60 minutes before procedure

NOTE: 1) Children 50 mg/kg (do not exceed adult dose)

                2) No second dose is required for adults or children

STANDARD REGIMEN FOR PATIENTS ALLERGIC TO AMOXICILLIN OR PENICILLIN

Rx	**Clindamycin 150 mg**

Disp   4 tablets

Sig   Take 4 tablets (600 mg) 30-60 minutes before procedure

OR

Rx	**Cephalexin 500 mg***

Disp   4 tablets

Sig   Take 4 tablets (2 g) 30-60 minutes before procedure

OR

PROPHYLACTIC ANTIBIOTIC COVERAGE FOR THE PREVENTION OF BACTERIAL ENDOCARDITIS

STANDARD REGIMEN FOR PATIENTS ALLERGIC TO AMOXICILLIN OR PENICILLIN *(continued)*

Rx	**Azithromycin 500 mg**
Disp	2 tablets
Sig	Take 1 tablet (500 mg) 30-60 minutes before procedure

OR

Rx	**Clarithromycin 250 mg**
Disp	2 tablets
Sig	Take 2 tablets (500 mg) 30-60 minutes before procedure

NOTE: Children's dosage (do not exceed adult dose)

Clindamycin 20 mg/kg
Cephalexin 50 mg/kg
Azithromycin 15 mg/kg
Clarithromycin 15 mg/kg

FOR PATIENTS UNABLE TO TAKE ORAL MEDICATION

Rx	**Ampicillin**

2 g I.V. or I.M. within 30 minutes before procedure

CHILDREN: 50 mg/kg I.V. or I.M. within 30 minutes before procedure

OR

PROPHYLACTIC ANTIBIOTIC COVERAGE FOR THE PREVENTION OF BACTERIAL ENDOCARDITIS

Rx   **Cefazolin* OR Ceftriaxone***

1 g I.V. or I.M. within 30 minutes before procedure

CHILDREN: 50 mg/kg I.V. or I.M. within 30 minutes before operation

FOR PATIENTS UNABLE TO TAKE ORAL MEDICATION AND ALLERGIC TO AMPICILLIN, AMOXICILLIN, PENICILLIN

Rx   **Clindamcyin**

600 mg I.V. within 30 minutes before procedure

CHILDREN: 20 mg/kg I.V. within 30 minutes before procedure

Rx   **Cefazolin* OR Ceftriaxone***

1 g I.V. or I.M. within 30 minutes before procedure

CHILDREN: 50 mg/kg I.V. or I.M. within 30 minutes before operation

* Cephalosporins should not be used in individuals with immediate-type hypersensitivity reaction (urticaria, angioedema, or anaphylaxis) to penicillin.

PROPHYLACTIC ANTIBIOTIC COVERAGE FOR PATIENTS WITH TOTAL JOINT REPLACEMENT

Current ADA and American Academy of Orthopedic Surgeons Joint Advisory Statement

Published July 2003, *JADA*, Vol 134, pp 895-899.

NOTE: Your patient with an artificial joint does not need antibiotic prophylaxis for any dental procedure unless they also meet one of the criteria below.

If patient's physician requests prophylaxis for dental procedure, but patient does not meet ADA/AAOS criteria for needing it, then physician should prescribe prophylaxis, patient takes it under their direction, and they come to you safe for dental procedures.

Patients at Potential Increased Risk of Hematogenous Total Joint Infection

Immunocompromised / Immunosuppressed Patients

Inflammatory arthropathies:
Rheumatoid arthritis
Systemic lupus erythematosus
Disease, drug, or radiation-induced immunosuppression

Other At-Risk Patients

Insulin-dependent (Type 1) diabetes
First 2 years following joint placement
Previous prosthetic joint infections
Malnourishment
Hemophilia

PROPHYLACTIC ANTIBIOTIC COVERAGE FOR PATIENTS WITH TOTAL JOINT REPLACEMENT

SUGGESTED ANTIBIOTIC REGIMENS

Rx	**Amoxicillin 500 mg**	(select ONE
	Cephalexin 500 mg	of these
	Cephradine 500 mg	antibiotics)

Disp   4 tablets

Sig   Take 4 tablets (2 g) 1 hour before procedure

IF PATIENT ALLERGIC TO PENICILLIN

Rx   **Clindamycin 150 mg**

Disp   4 tablets

Sig   Take 4 tablets (600 mg) 1 hour before procedure

IF PATIENT UNABLE TO TAKE ORAL MEDICATION

Rx   **Cefazolin**

Sig   1 g or Ampicillin 2 g I.M. or I.V., 1 hour before procedure

IF PATIENT ALLERGIC TO PENICILLIN AND UNABLE TO TAKE ORAL MEDICATIONS

Rx   **Clindamycin**

Sig   600 mg I.V., 1 hour before procedure

NOTES

9) TOBACCO CESSATION

Wellbutrin SR

Chantix

Nicotine Replacement Therapy

TOBACCO CESSATION

As a healthcare provider, you care. Tobacco use causes multiple health problems. You can help. You can intervene; it takes only 3 minutes.

Ask about your patient's tobacco use

Advise to quit

Assess for readiness to quit

Assist if ready to quit (drugs, substitutes below)

Arrange for follow-up care (the patient should arrange for counseling - it helps a lot)

Rx	**Zyban (Wellbutrin SR) 150 mg**
Disp	60 tablets
Sig	Starting 1 week from quit date, take 1 tablet per day for 3 days, then take 2 tablets per day (at least 8 hours apart) for 7-12 weeks

OR

Rx	**Chantix 1 mg**
Disp	60 tablets
Sig	Starting 1 week before quit date, take 1/2 tablet per day for 3 days, then 1/2 tablet 2 times per day (at least 8 hours apart) for 4 days, then take 1 tablet 2 times per day (at least 8 hours apart) for 12 weeks

TOBACCO CESSATION

Nicotine Replacement Therapy (eg, **Nicorette** gum, patches, or inhalers) is available OTC and can be used, but alone it is less effective than the drugs on the previous page.

Tobacco cessation is a complex psychological and physiological process. Though a dentist has a duty to the patient's overall health, once they have done the 5 A's listed on the previous page, the dentist may elect to refer the patient to a physician for pharmacologic intervention.

Tobacco Cessation Websites:

http://www1.umn.edu/perio/tobacco/didactic.html

(comprehensive dental site for all aspects of quitting, including patient handouts)

http://www.askadviserefer.org/

(an excellent resource from the ADHA for everyone in the dental office)

http://www.ctcinfo.org/

(a very comprehensive site for everyone - healthcare professionals and smokers)

NOTES

NOTES

NOTES

Lexi-Comp ON-HAND for Dentistry

Lexi-Comp ON-HAND for Dentistry is our top-rated software that provides instant access to point-of-care information on a handheld device. Advanced navigation tools make it easy to find the right information when you need it the most. Updates to our content are available on a daily basis, ensuring you always have the most up-to-date clinical information at your fingertips.

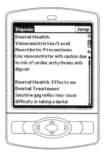

Dental Lexi-Drugs®, our master database of drug information specific to dentistry, includes information on over 7500 drugs. These monographs contain up to 30 fields of information, including the following key fields:

- ■ U.S. Brand Names and Generic Names
- ■ Special Alerts
- ■ Use
- ■ Local Anesthetic/Vasoconstrictor Precautions
- ■ Effects on Dental Treatment
- ■ Dental Dosing for Selected Drug Classifications
- ■ Adverse Effects, Contraindications, Warnings/Precautions
- ■ Drug Interactions
- ■ Dental Comment

For more information or to place an order:
Call: 1-800-837-5394 or visit: www.lexi.com/lddb

Lexi-Comp ON-DESKTOP for Dentistry

Lexi-Comp ON-DESKTOP for Dentistry is the ultimate solution for
Complete Medication Management, allowing you
to store and edit office and patient medication
regimens. Our complete library of databases is
downloaded to your desktop computer, or
hosted on your network server, eliminating
the need for a constant Internet connection.
Unlimited updates, available during your
subscription period, are scheduled to meet
your needs and retrieved via the Internet.

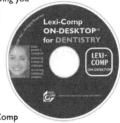

Elevate the standard of patient care and help
protect your practice from liability with Lexi-Comp
ON-DESKTOP for Dentistry.

With Lexi-Comp ON-DESKTOP for Dentistry:

■ Obtain instant DENTAL ALERTS warning of medications that will influence
treatment or cause harmful effects to the patient
- o Effects on Dental Treatment
- o Effects on Bleeding
- o Vasoconstrictor/Local Anesthetic Precautions
- o Dental Comment

■ Store your patient medication lists to help ensure safe treatment plans

■ Easily implement Drug Interaction Analysis into your office workflow
- o Supplemental Patient Drug Form provided (English/Spanish)

■ Compare therapeutic categories to your patient drug regimens to select
the most appropriate medication

■ Access over 1,000 color photographs and radiographs

■ Review nearly 12,000 drugs in the Drug ID module

■ Print medication leaflets for your patients in 18 languages

For more information or to place an order:
Call: 1-800-837-5394 or visit: www.lexi.com/lddb

Lexi-Comp ONLINE for Dentistry

This powerful Internet-based application provides **real-time** access to all Lexi-Comp dentistry knowledge areas. Simply enter a user name and password on a computer with Internet connectivity and navigate to any content area within three mouse clicks! Drug monographs can be accessed directly from a condition or procedure using built-in links. Detailed photographs and radiographs are included.

- Obtain instant DENTAL ALERTS warning of medications that will influence treatment or cause harmful effects to the patient
    - o Effects on Dental Treatment
    - o Effects on Bleeding
    - o Vasoconstrictor/Local Anesthetic Precautions
    - o Dental Comment

- Easily implement Drug Interaction Analysis into your office workflow
    - o Supplemental Patient Drug Form provided (English/Spanish)

- Compare therapeutic categories to your patient drug regimens to select the most appropriate medication

- Access over 1,000 color photographs and radiographs

- Review nearly 12,000 drugs in the Drug ID module

- Print medication leaflets for your patients in 18 languages

- Utilize Web Search and expand your search capabilities to other qualified health web sites

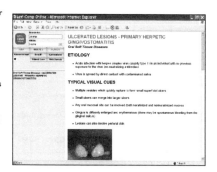

For more information or to place an order:
Call: 1-800-837-5394 or visit: www.lexi.com/lddb

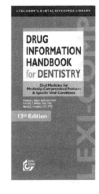

Lexi-Comp's DENTISTRY SOLUTIONS

At Lexi-Comp, we understand that no two patients are alike, presenting individual challenges for optimizing treatment. These challenges require a wide range of resources that are reliable, clinically-relevant, and available at the point-of-care in a variety of formats.

Our Dentistry knowledge areas include:
- Drug Information for Dentistry
- Drug Interactions
- Natural Therapeutics
- Dental Implants
- Clinical Endodontics
- Clinical Periodontics
- Oral Soft Tissue Diseases
- Oral Hard Tissue Diseases
- Oral Surgery
- Dental Office Medical Emergencies
- Financial Integrity in the Dental Office
- Employee Embezzlement & Fraud
- Patient Education
- Drug Identification
- Complementary licensed PDA resources:
    - Stedman's Medical Dictionary for the Health Professions and Nursing
    - The 5-Minute Clinical Consult
    - Harrison's Practice

Our Dentistry information is available in a variety of electronic formats and in our reference library of dental titles.

For more information or to place an order:
Call: 1-800-837-5394 or visit: www.lexi.com/lddb

IMPROVING POINT-OF-CARE DECISIONS

Access More. Provide More.

I am delighted that you have found my little dental drug booklet useful (at least, I hope it was useful). And thank you for your help over the years. The booklet has grown based on your practical, practice-oriented suggestions. If you have any edits, suggestions, or topics you would like added, please let me know at my e-mail address, by snail-mail, or by phone. I will try to incorporate the information into next year's edition.

Thank you.

Peter J.

Peter L. Jacobsen, PhD, DDS
Professor, Dept. of Pathology and Medicine
University of the Pacific
Arthur A. Dugoni School of Dentistry
2155 Webster Street, Room 400
San Francisco, California 94115
415-929-6609
415-921-0484 (fax)
pgjacobs@pacbell.net
www.peterjacobsen.com (website)